Dr. Barbara
Parasite Cleanse

The Nutritional Guide for Individuals to
Treat and Eliminate Parasites and
Parasitic Infections with Natural Barbara
O'Neill Remedies,Diet and Method

ISBN 978-1-304-01857-1
Brynlee Jannika

TABLE OF CONTENT

CHAPTER 1

INTRODUCTION

A. Introduction to Parasitic Infections

Infections caused by parasites are quite common and can impact individuals of all ages, genders, and geographical locations. Parasites are living organisms that thrive by taking advantage of a host organism, obtaining nutrients at the host's expense. They come in a wide range of sizes, from tiny protozoa to larger worms, and their presence can cause a variety of health issues.

There are various types of infections that can be caused by parasites, including intestinal worms, protozoa, and ectoparasites. Various methods of transmission exist for these organisms to infiltrate the body, including ingestion of contaminated substances, insect-induced punctures, or contact with tainted surfaces.

The symptoms of infections caused by parasites can vary greatly, depending on the specific type of infection and how severe it is. Typical signs and symptoms encompass various gastrointestinal problems like diarrhea, abdominal discomfort, and bloating; overall symptoms like fatigue, weight loss, and anemia; and skin-related symptoms such as itching and rashes. In severe cases, infections caused by parasites can result in long-term health issues and weaken the immune system.

B. The Significance of Natural Treatment Methods

Treatment for parasitic infections typically involves the use of pharmaceutical medications, which can be effective but may also have potential side effects. These medications may occasionally result in resistance, which can make treating future infections more challenging. In addition, they may fail to address the root causes that make the body vulnerable to parasites in the first place.

Alternative treatment methods provide a comprehensive approach to dealing with parasitic infections. These methods focus on eradicating parasites while also enhancing the body's immune system, promoting gut health, and preventing future infestations. Alternative therapies are typically more gentle on the body, minimizing the potential for adverse reactions and supporting overall well-being.

Some advantages of utilizing natural treatment methods are:

1. Reducing Side Effects: Natural remedies, including specific foods, herbs, and lifestyle adjustments, are generally gentler on the body in comparison to pharmaceutical drugs.
2. Preventing Drug Resistance: Through the implementation of diverse natural treatments, the likelihood of parasites developing resistance can be minimized.
3. Promoting Overall Health: Embracing natural methods often entails making adjustments to one's diet and lifestyle, which can have a positive impact on overall health and well-being.
4. Identifying Underlying Factors: These treatments can assist in recognizing and resolving factors that contribute to vulnerability to parasitic infections, such as inadequate nutrition, compromised immune system, and exposure to polluted surroundings.

 C. Introduction to Barbara O'Neill and Her Approach

Barbara O'Neill is a highly respected naturopath and health educator recognized for her extensive knowledge in natural healing methods. With years of expertise in the realm of natural health, Barbara has assisted numerous individuals in conquering a range of health obstacles using her comprehensive approach.

Barbara O'Neill's approach to addressing parasites centers around utilizing nourishing foods, beneficial herbs, and lifestyle adjustments that enhance the body's innate capacity to heal and protect itself from infections. Her approach is based on the understanding that the body has the ability to heal itself with the right support and resources.

Philosophy and Principles: Barbara O'Neill's approach is guided by a set of core principles:

1. Embracing Nature's Solutions: She strongly supports the utilization of natural remedies, including specific foods and herbs with a long history of effectively combating parasitic infections.
2. Dietary Adjustments: Barbara highlights the significance of maintaining a well-rounded diet that is abundant in nourishing elements to enhance the immune system and foster a healthy gut.
3. Detoxification: She strongly advocates for the benefits of detoxification in purifying the body from harmful substances, including the toxins

produced by unwanted organisms.

4. Lifestyle Modifications: Barbara emphasizes the importance of making changes to one's lifestyle, including practicing better hygiene and managing stress, in order to prevent and effectively manage infections caused by parasites.

5. Education and Empowerment: A crucial element of Barbara's approach involves providing individuals with knowledge about their health and encouraging them to actively manage their well-being.

Important Aspects of Barbara O'Neill's Approach:

1. Foods with Natural Antiparasitic Properties: Barbara suggests adding certain foods to your diet that naturally combat parasites. Certain foods, such as raw garlic, onions, pumpkin seeds, pineapple, and papaya seeds, have been recognized for their potential to help eliminate parasites and promote a healthy gut.

2. Natural Remedies: Some herbs have proven to be highly effective in fighting against parasites. Barbara frequently recommends the use of herbs like wormwood, black walnut hull, and cloves due to their strong antiparasitic properties. These herbs can be utilized in a variety of ways, such as brewing them

into teas, creating tinctures, or encapsulating them.

3. Detoxification Protocols: Cleansing the body is essential for eliminating harmful organisms and their byproducts. Barbara promotes the use of detox programs, including juice fasting, herbal detox teas, and colon cleansing, to assist the body's natural detoxification processes.

4. Staying properly hydrated is crucial for eliminating toxins and promoting overall well-being. In addition, including foods that are rich in probiotics, like yogurt and kefir, can help rebalance the gut's beneficial bacteria, creating an environment that is less favorable for parasites.

5. Prevention Strategies: Barbara highlights the significance of taking preventive measures to lower the chances of getting infected by parasites. It is important to maintain good hygiene, ensure the safety of food and water sources, and strengthen the immune system with a nutrient-rich diet and regular exercise.

Barbara O'Neill's approach to addressing and getting rid of parasitic infections is based on natural healing principles that prioritize assisting the body's inherent healing capabilities. By incorporating targeted foods, herbs, dietary changes, and lifestyle adjustments, her approach offers a complete and holistic approach to addressing parasitic infections while fostering overall health and wellness.

CHAPTER 2

Understanding Parasites

A. Common Types of Parasites

There are different types of parasites that can cause infections, each with their own characteristics and ways of infecting their hosts. Gaining knowledge about these organisms is crucial for successful treatment and prevention. In this exploration, we delve into three primary categories: intestinal worms, protozoa, and ectoparasites.

1. Dealing with Intestinal Worms

Intestinal worms, or helminths, are a prevalent type of parasite that can affect humans. They have the ability to reside in the digestive tract and various other areas of the body, resulting in a variety of health problems.

- Roundworms, also known as nematodes, are elongated, unsegmented worms that have the ability to inhabit various tissues, including the intestines. There are a few types of roundworms that can cause infections in humans. One of them is Ascaris lumbricoides, which is responsible for ascariasis. Another is

Enterobius vermicularis, which is commonly known for causing pinworm infections. Common symptoms can manifest as abdominal pain, diarrhea, malnutrition, and respiratory issues when the larvae migrate through the lungs.

- Tapeworms (Cestodes): Tapeworms are elongated, segmented worms that can reach impressive lengths. They firmly attach to the walls of the intestines using their scolex, or head, and then proceed to absorb nutrients through their skin. Some well-known species are Taenia saginata (beef tapeworm) and Taenia solium (pork tapeworm). Tapeworm infections may lead to digestive disturbances, weight loss, and in more severe cases, cysticercosis, where larvae develop cysts in tissues such as muscles and the brain.

- Flukes (Trematodes): Flukes are flat, leaf-shaped worms that commonly reside in the liver, lungs, or blood vessels. Some of the most well-known flukes are the Schistosoma species, which are responsible for causing schistosomiasis. The symptoms can differ based on the specific species and where the infection occurs, but they might encompass fever, abdominal discomfort, diarrhea, and gradual organ deterioration.

2. Protozoa

Protozoa, those tiny single-celled organisms, have the potential to wreak havoc on our health, especially when it comes to the gastrointestinal and urogenital systems. They have a remarkable ability to multiply quickly and outsmart the host's immune system using a range of tactics.

- Giardia lamblia: Giardia is a flagellated protozoan that causes giardiasis, a common intestinal infection. Transmission occurs through the consumption of contaminated water and food. Common symptoms may include diarrhea, abdominal cramps, bloating, nausea, and malabsorption, which can result in weight loss and malnutrition.

- The protozoan known as Entamoeba histolytica is responsible for causing amoebiasis, a condition that can lead to symptoms such as severe diarrhea, abdominal pain, and the formation of liver abscesses. It is transmitted through the consumption of cysts found in unclean water or contaminated food. Severe infections can result in extensive harm to the intestinal lining and other tissues.

- Plasmodium species are responsible for causing malaria, a highly severe and prevalent parasitic disease. Transmitted by Anopheles mosquitoes, malaria can cause symptoms such as fever, chills, anemia, and organ failure. The most harmful species, Plasmodium falciparum, has the potential to cause cerebral malaria, a condition that can be fatal if not treated.

3. External Parasites

There are certain types of parasites that thrive on the host's body, specifically on the surface, and they have a tendency to feed on blood or skin cells. They can be quite bothersome, causing discomfort, skin irritation, and even transmitting other infectious agents.

- Lice: These pesky creatures are tiny insects that invade the hair and skin. Head lice are a frequent occurrence among school-aged children, resulting in uncomfortable itching and irritation of the scalp. Body lice, specifically Pediculus humanus corporis, are commonly found on clothing and have the potential to spread diseases like typhus.

- Fleas: These tiny, wingless insects have a rather unpleasant habit of feasting on the blood of mammals and birds. They can result in itching, provoke allergic reactions, and spread diseases such as plague (Yersinia pestis) and typhus (Rickettsia typhi).

- Mites: Certain types of mites, like Sarcoptes scabiei, can lead to scabies, a skin condition that manifests as severe itching and a rash. Scabies mites burrow into the skin to lay eggs, which can cause inflammation and potentially lead to secondary bacterial infections.

B. Signs of Parasitic Infections

The symptoms of infections caused by parasites can differ greatly, depending on the specific parasite, where the infection is located, and how severe the infestation is. Typical signs and symptoms may include:

- Gastrointestinal Symptoms: Diarrhea, abdominal pain, bloating, nausea, vomiting, and changes in appetite are common symptoms associated with intestinal parasites.
- General Symptoms: Fatigue, weakness, unexplained weight loss, and anemia may manifest as parasites consume the host's nutrients.
- Skin Troubles: Itching, rashes, and skin lesions often accompany ectoparasite

infections and certain protozoan
infections.
- Respiratory Symptoms: Experience
coughing, wheezing, and shortness of
breath as a result of parasites migrating
through the lungs.
- Symptoms of the Nervous System:
Headaches, seizures, and cognitive
impairment can occur due to parasites
affecting the central nervous system, as
seen in cases like cerebral malaria or
neurocysticercosis.

C. Risk Factors and Transmission of
Infections

Gaining knowledge about the risk factors
and ways in which parasitic infections are
spread is essential for effectively
preventing and managing these diseases.

Factors that Increase the Risk

- Lack of Proper Sanitation and Hygiene:
Insufficient sanitation facilities and
inadequate personal hygiene practices
heighten the chances of coming into
contact with parasites through
contaminated water, food, and surfaces.
- Geographical Location: Residing in or
visiting regions with a high occurrence of
parasitic infections, such as tropical and
subtropical areas, can elevate the risk.

- People with weakened immune systems, such as those with HIV/AIDS, malnutrition, or chronic diseases, are more vulnerable to parasitic infections due to their compromised immune systems.
- Occupation and Lifestyle: Certain occupations and activities that entail frequent interaction with soil, animals, or untreated water, such as farming, fishing, and swimming, can heighten the risk of exposure to parasites.

Transmission Routes

- Transmission through Ingestion: Numerous parasites can be transmitted when individuals consume water or food that has been contaminated. Giardia, Entamoeba histolytica, and various intestinal worms can be contracted through this method.
- Direct Contact: Coming into direct contact with contaminated soil or surfaces can result in infections caused by certain parasites, such as hookworms and schistosomes.
- Transmission through Vectors: Certain parasites, such as Plasmodium (malaria) and filarial worms, are spread through insect bites from vectors like mosquitoes and flies.
- Transmission between individuals: Parasites like lice, scabies mites, and

pinworms have the ability to spread when there is close personal contact or when personal items such as clothing and bedding are shared.
- Transmission through Ingestion: Infections caused by certain parasites, such as Giardia and Entamoeba histolytica, can occur when individuals consume contaminated hands, food, or objects that have come into contact with feces.

Through a comprehensive understanding of the various types of parasites, the ability to identify the symptoms they induce, and a heightened awareness of the factors that increase the risk of infection and the ways in which parasites are transmitted, individuals can adopt a proactive approach to effectively prevent and manage parasitic infections. This understanding forms the basis of the natural treatment approaches recommended by Barbara O'Neill, which focus on eradicating parasites while promoting the body's overall well-being and strength.

CHAPTER 3

Foods to Eliminate Parasites

Using certain foods that have properties to fight against parasitic infections can be a highly effective and natural approach. These foods can effectively get rid of parasites and make it difficult for them to survive, reducing the risk of future infestations. Here, we explore five powerful foods known for their ability to combat parasites: raw garlic, onions, pumpkin seeds, pineapple, and papaya seeds.

A. Antiparasitic Foods
 1. Fresh Garlic

Raw garlic is an incredibly potent natural solution for getting rid of parasites. Throughout history, this substance has been valued by different societies for its therapeutic qualities.

- Active Compounds: Garlic contains allicin and ajoene, which possess potent properties against parasites, fungi, bacteria, and viruses. When garlic is crushed or chopped, it releases compounds that have a powerful ability to eliminate parasites.

- How it Works: Allicin interferes with the parasites' metabolism and causes harm to their cell membranes, hindering their ability to survive and reproduce. In addition, garlic can stimulate the production of digestive enzymes that aid in the removal of parasites from the gastrointestinal tract.
- Tip: For optimal effectiveness against parasites, try consuming raw garlic on an empty stomach. To fully unlock the potential of garlic, it is recommended to finely chop or crush a few cloves and allow them to rest for a short period of time. This will activate the allicin compound, enhancing its beneficial properties. You have the option of combining it with honey or diluting it in a small amount of water to enhance its taste.

 2. Onions

Onions, which are closely related to garlic, have powerful properties that can help fight against infections caused by parasites.

- Active Compounds: Onions possess sulfur compounds like sulfoxides and thiosulfinates, known for their antimicrobial and antiparasitic properties.
- Mode of Action: The sulfur compounds found in onions have the ability to

eliminate parasites and hinder their development. Onions also help to stimulate the digestive system, supporting the body in eliminating harmful organisms and their toxins.
- Usage: Raw onions are highly effective for combating parasites. They can be included in salads, salsas, or enjoyed as juice. Regular consumption of a mixture of onion juice and water can be beneficial in addressing the issue of unwanted organisms. Make sure the onions are fresh and raw to maintain the integrity of their beneficial compounds.

3. Pumpkin Seeds

Pumpkin seeds have long been used as a natural remedy to eliminate intestinal parasites, specifically tapeworms and roundworms.

- Effective Ingredients: Pumpkin seeds contain cucurbitacin, an amino acid that immobilizes parasites, facilitating their removal from the body. They are also packed with zinc and other essential nutrients that help boost the immune system.
- Mechanism of Action: Cucurbitacin induces paralysis in the worms, inhibiting their ability to cling to the intestinal walls. This paralysis enables the natural

removal of the parasites through bowel movements.
- Instructions: Eat a few raw, unshelled pumpkin seeds when you haven't eaten anything. You have the option to grind them into a fine powder and incorporate them into your beverages or yogurt. To enhance the effectiveness, try combining pumpkin seeds with other foods or herbs known for their antiparasitic properties, like garlic or coconut oil.

 4. Pineapple

Pineapple is not just a tasty fruit, but it also possesses natural properties that can help combat parasites, thanks to its enzyme content.

- Active Compounds: Pineapple contains bromelain, a powerful enzyme that aids in the breakdown of proteins and the dissolution of parasites and their eggs.
- How it Works: Bromelain has the ability to disrupt the protective layer of parasites, rendering them more susceptible to the digestive enzymes and the immune system. Pineapple also possesses properties that can aid in reducing the symptoms of parasitic infections by reducing inflammation.
- Usage: Fresh pineapple is highly effective for antiparasitic purposes. Incorporate fresh pineapple slices or

fresh pineapple juice into your daily routine. Steer clear of canned pineapple or juice that contains added sugars, as these can reduce the fruit's beneficial properties.

5. Seeds from the Papaya Fruit

Papaya seeds have been found to be highly effective in naturally getting rid of intestinal parasites, specifically roundworms and tapeworms.

- Active Compounds: Papaya seeds contain enzymes that have potent properties against parasites. They also contain alkaloids that have properties to eliminate parasites.
- Mode of Action: Papain degrades the proteins found in parasites and their eggs, leading to their effective elimination. The seeds also aid in digestion and support the elimination of parasites through bowel movements.
- Purpose: To utilize the potential of papaya seeds for combating parasites, simply grind a tablespoon of fresh papaya seeds and combine them with honey, water, or smoothies. Take this mixture on an empty stomach every day for a week. Alternatively, the seeds can be consumed whole, although their intense, peppery flavor might not appeal to everyone.

Adding these foods to your diet can help you naturally fight off parasitic infections. Raw garlic, onions, pumpkin seeds, pineapple, and papaya seeds possess distinct properties that can disrupt and eliminate parasites, thereby aiding the body's natural defenses. Incorporating these foods into your diet can support a well-functioning digestive system and reduce the risk of future infestations.

B. Fermented Foods
Fermented foods contain probiotics, which are beneficial bacteria that support a healthy gut microbiome. An optimal gut microbiome plays a vital role in bolstering the body's immune system and enhancing digestion, which in turn helps protect against parasitic infections. Here, we delve into three fermented foods—sauerkraut, kimchi, and kombucha—that have been found to be beneficial for gut health and can help with getting rid of parasites.

1. Fermented cabbage

Sauerkraut is a delightful creation made from fermented cabbage, packed with a plethora of beneficial probiotics, vitamins, and minerals. For centuries, people have turned to this natural remedy for its numerous health benefits and its ability to promote a healthy digestive system.

- Beneficial Bacteria: Sauerkraut contains a rich amount of Lactobacillus species, which play a crucial role in restoring the natural balance of the gut microbiome. These beneficial microorganisms have the ability to prevent the proliferation of harmful microorganisms, including those that can cause harm to the body.
- Nutrient Profile: Sauerkraut provides a range of essential vitamins and minerals, including vitamins C and K, iron, manganese, and dietary fiber. Consuming Vitamin C can enhance the immune system, enabling the body to combat infections effectively. Additionally, including fiber in your diet can promote regular bowel movements, which can assist in eliminating parasites.
- Mechanism of Action: The probiotics in sauerkraut work by creating an acidic environment in the gut that is not ideal for parasites to thrive. Additionally, they boost the production of natural antibodies and activate the immune response, which creates a less favorable environment for parasites to survive.
- Recommendation: Consider adding a small portion of sauerkraut to your daily meals. It can be included in salads, sandwiches, or enjoyed as a side dish. Make sure to select raw, unpasteurized sauerkraut to preserve the beneficial bacteria.

2. Kimchi

Kimchi is a classic Korean delicacy that showcases the art of fermentation. It features a harmonious blend of vegetables, including cabbage and radishes, enhanced by a medley of flavors like garlic, ginger, and chili peppers. Renowned for its powerful probiotic content and numerous health advantages.

- Beneficial Bacteria: Similar to sauerkraut, kimchi contains a generous amount of Lactobacillus species and other helpful bacteria. These probiotics support the maintenance of a healthy balance of gut flora and hinder the growth of harmful organisms.
- Nutrient Profile: Kimchi is rich in essential vitamins and minerals, along with dietary fiber and beneficial antioxidants. The vegetables and seasonings used in kimchi offer a variety of nutrients that help maintain overall health and support immune function.
- Mechanism of Action: The fermentation process of kimchi generates lactic acid, which aids in reducing the pH of the gut. This creates an unfavorable environment for parasites to thrive. The probiotics also help to improve digestion and boost the body's natural defense mechanisms.

- Usage: Kimchi is versatile and can be used in various ways, such as a condiment, side dish, or as an ingredient in soups and stews. Incorporating a regular portion of kimchi into your diet can contribute to the well-being of your digestive system and enhance your body's natural defense against harmful organisms. Just like sauerkraut, opt for raw, unpasteurized kimchi to make sure you get those beneficial live probiotics.

 3. Kombucha

Kombucha has become quite popular due to its probiotic content and the health benefits it offers. It is created through the process of fermenting sweetened tea with a symbiotic culture of bacteria and yeast (SCOBY).

- Beneficial Microorganisms: Kombucha is rich in a variety of strains of helpful bacteria and yeasts, such as Lactobacillus and Bifidobacterium species. These beneficial bacteria promote a balanced gut microbiome and hinder the proliferation of detrimental organisms.
- Nutrient Profile: Kombucha contains a variety of beneficial compounds including B vitamins, antioxidants, and organic acids like acetic acid and gluconic acid. These compounds possess antimicrobial

properties and can aid in the body's detoxification processes.

- Mechanism of Action: The organic acids in kombucha help create an environment in the gut that is less favorable for parasites. The beneficial bacteria in kombucha also compete with harmful organisms for resources and adhesion sites in the gut, which aids in the prevention of infections.

- Recommendation: Incorporate a daily glass of kombucha into your routine for optimal probiotic benefits, preferably on an empty stomach. Begin with a modest quantity and slowly raise the consumption to prevent any digestive discomfort. Choose raw, unpasteurized kombucha that is free from added sugars or artificial flavors to guarantee the presence of live probiotics.

Adding fermented foods such as sauerkraut, kimchi, and kombucha to your diet can greatly improve gut health and help eliminate unwanted organisms. These foods contain beneficial bacteria that promote a healthy gut, prevent the growth of harmful organisms, and boost the immune system. Consistently incorporating fermented foods into your diet can create an inhospitable environment in the gut, which can be beneficial in preventing and managing infections caused by parasites.

C. Probiotic-Rich Foods

Consuming foods that are rich in probiotics is vital for maintaining a healthy gut microbiome, which is crucial for preventing and managing infections caused by parasites. These foods are packed with helpful bacteria that promote gut health, strengthen the immune system, and aid in the removal of unwanted organisms. Unsweetened yogurt and kefir are two great sources of probiotics. Let's delve into the advantages and see how they can assist in eradicating parasites.

1. Unsweetened Yogurt

Yogurt is a popular food that is made by fermenting milk with live bacterial cultures, known for their beneficial properties. It is a highly adaptable food that can be seamlessly integrated into any diet.

- Beneficial Bacteria: Unsweetened yogurt is rich in probiotics, including Lactobacillus bulgaricus, Streptococcus thermophilus, Lactobacillus acidophilus, and Bifidobacterium bifidum. These probiotics are beneficial for promoting and sustaining a harmonious gut microbiome.
- Nutrient Profile: Yogurt contains a variety of essential nutrients, including

protein, calcium, vitamins B2 (riboflavin), B12, potassium, and magnesium. These nutrients help maintain overall health and support the immune system, enhancing the body's ability to fight off infections.

- Mechanism of Action: The probiotics in yogurt work by colonizing the gut and creating an unfavorable environment for unwanted organisms. They achieve this by producing lactic acid, which helps to lower the pH of the intestine. The acidic environment hinders the development and existence of parasites. In addition, probiotics can improve the gut's barrier function, which helps to prevent harmful pathogens from attaching to the walls of the intestines.

- Usage: For optimal results, opt for plain, unsweetened yogurt that contains live and active cultures. Many sweetened or flavored yogurts on the market today are made with added sugars and artificial ingredients, which can reduce the potential probiotic advantages they offer. Make sure to incorporate a serving of yogurt into your daily diet, whether you enjoy it on its own or as part of a meal. It can be incorporated into smoothies, utilized as a foundation for dips, or savored alongside fresh fruits and nuts.

 Tips for a Healthy Breakfast: - Mix yogurt with fresh berries, a handful of

nuts, and a drizzle of honey for a nutritious start to your day.
- Smoothies: Mix yogurt with your preferred fruits and vegetables to create a smoothie packed with probiotics.
- Salad Dressings: Incorporate yogurt into your salad dressings for a creamy and flavorful twist. Combine it with herbs, garlic, lemon juice, and olive oil to create a delicious dressing.
- Dips: Create nutritious dips by mixing yogurt with cucumber, garlic, and dill to achieve a revitalizing tzatziki sauce.

2. Kefir

Kefir is a delightful fermented milk drink with its origins in the majestic Caucasus Mountains. The flavor is zesty and the texture has a subtle fizziness, thanks to the fermentation process.

- Beneficial Microorganisms: Kefir is rich in a variety of helpful bacteria and yeasts, such as Lactobacillus kefiranofaciens, Lactobacillus acidophilus, Bifidobacterium bifidum, and Saccharomyces kefir. Kefir contains a wider range of probiotics compared to yogurt, offering a greater diversity of beneficial microorganisms.
- Nutrient Profile: Similar to yogurt, kefir contains a variety of essential nutrients including protein, calcium, B vitamins, magnesium, and phosphorus. In addition,

it contains bioactive compounds like peptides and polysaccharides that have properties that promote good health.

- Mechanism of Action: Kefir's probiotics work by replenishing the gut with helpful bacteria, which improves the diversity and strength of the gut microbiome. The probiotics generate organic acids and antimicrobial compounds that hinder the proliferation of parasites and other harmful microorganisms. Kefir also enhances digestion and strengthens the immune system, facilitating the body's ability to fight off infections.

- Usage: Enjoy kefir as a refreshing beverage or incorporate it into your favorite recipes such as smoothies, salad dressings, and marinades. Similar to yogurt, opting for plain, unsweetened kefir is recommended to steer clear of any additional sugars or artificial additives. If you're new to kefir, it's best to start with a small amount. The high probiotic content of kefir can sometimes lead to digestive adjustments.

Tips for Incorporation: - Smoothies: Mix kefir with a variety of fruits, vegetables, and a hint of honey to create a delicious and healthy smoothie.

- Salad Dressings: Enhance the nutritional value of your salad dressings by combining kefir with a delightful blend of herbs, mustard, lemon juice, and olive oil.

- Marinades: Incorporate kefir into your cooking routine by using it as a flavorful marinade for meats and vegetables. The acidity of this ingredient aids in the tenderization of the protein and imparts a distinct taste.

- On Its Own: Indulge in a glass of kefir for a beverage that is rich in probiotics, perfect for aiding digestion, particularly after meals.

Adding probiotic-rich foods such as unsweetened yogurt and kefir to your diet can greatly improve gut health and help eliminate unwanted organisms. The helpful bacteria found in these foods contribute to a healthy gut microbiome, creating an unfavorable environment for unwanted organisms and enhancing the immune system. Incorporating these foods into your diet can help boost your overall health and strengthen your body's natural defenses against infections caused by parasites.

D. Hydration and Detoxification

Proper hydration and detoxification are essential for maintaining optimal health and preventing and eliminating infections caused by parasites. Staying properly hydrated aids in eliminating harmful substances and unwanted organisms from the body, while incorporating targeted detoxification methods can further amplify this benefit. This section delves into the significance of water and the advantages of lemon water in enhancing hydration and detoxification.

1. The Significance of Water

Water is vital for sustaining life and plays a crucial role in the functioning of every cell and organ in the body. It is crucial for a range of physiological processes, such as digestion, circulation, temperature regulation, and waste elimination.

- Optimal Cellular Function: Ensuring proper hydration is essential for cells to function at their best. Water plays a vital role in cellular metabolism, facilitating the transportation of nutrients and the elimination of metabolic waste products. Ensuring adequate hydration is essential for preserving the integrity of cellular membranes and promoting optimal enzymatic activities, which are vital for overall well-being.
- Detoxification and Waste Removal: The kidneys play a crucial role in filtering blood and eliminating waste products and toxins from the body. Ensuring sufficient water intake helps maintain optimal kidney function and aids in the body's natural detoxification process by

encouraging urine production. This aids in eliminating parasites and the harmful substances they produce.

- Optimal Digestive Function: Water plays a crucial role in supporting the efficient digestion and absorption of nutrients by promoting the breakdown of food and the smooth movement of waste through the digestive system. Staying properly hydrated is essential for maintaining regular bowel movements and creating an unfavorable environment for parasites to thrive. Regular bowel movements are important for eliminating parasites and their eggs from the body, and water plays a crucial role in this process.

- Immune Function: Water plays a crucial role in maintaining a healthy immune system by promoting proper circulation of lymph, a fluid that contains white blood cells, throughout the body. This circulation is crucial for identifying and eliminating pathogens, such as parasites. Proper hydration is essential for keeping the mucous membranes in the respiratory and gastrointestinal tracts healthy, as they act as protective barriers against infections.

 Suggestions for Maintaining Proper Hydration:
- Stay Hydrated: It is important to maintain proper hydration by drinking an

adequate amount of water every day. Aim for at least eight 8-ounce glasses of water, or adjust based on factors such as your activity level, climate, and personal requirements.

- Keep an eye on your urine: An excellent way to determine if you are properly hydrated is by observing the color of your urine. When it comes to urine color, a pale yellow hue usually suggests that you're well-hydrated, whereas a darker yellow or amber color may be a sign of dehydration.

- Stay Hydrated: Make sure to have a water bottle with you at all times to help you stay hydrated throughout the day.

- Stay properly hydrated before, during, and after exercise: Staying properly hydrated is crucial when engaging in physical activity. Sweating during exercise leads to increased water loss, making it essential to drink water before, during, and after your workout.

2. Refreshing Citrus Infusion

Drinking lemon water can be a refreshing and beneficial method to increase your body's hydration levels and support detoxification processes. Enhance the health benefits of water by incorporating the invigorating freshness of lemon juice, which can aid in the removal of unwanted organisms.

- Nutrient Content: Lemons contain a significant amount of vitamin C, which is known for its antioxidant properties that can boost the immune system and counteract the effects of free radicals. They also include trace amounts of potassium, magnesium, and vitamin B6.
- Balancing pH: Despite their tangy flavor, lemons help balance the body's pH levels once metabolized. Keeping the body's pH balance in check can help create an environment that is less hospitable to parasites and other harmful microorganisms.
- Enhances Digestion: Lemon water promotes the production of digestive juices, such as bile, which supports the digestion and absorption of nutrients. It can assist in reducing digestive problems like bloating, indigestion, and constipation, which can create a favorable environment for unwelcome guests.
- Promoting Liver Health: Lemon water aids in supporting liver function by stimulating the production of enzymes that assist in detoxifying the liver. The liver has a vital function in removing harmful substances and disease-causing agents from the bloodstream. By improving liver function, lemon water aids the body in more effectively eliminating parasites.

- Hydration and Satiety: Adding lemon to water can enhance its taste, which may help to increase water consumption. Ensuring adequate hydration is crucial for supporting optimal bodily functions, including the important process of detoxification. Drinking lemon water can also contribute to a sense of satiety, potentially aiding in portion control and weight management.

 Here's a simple way to prepare and enjoy lemon water: Just squeeze the juice of half a lemon into a glass of warm or room-temperature water. Start your day off right by drinking it first thing in the morning to boost your metabolism and stay hydrated throughout the day.
- Refreshing Beverage: Enhance the flavor of your water by adding slices of lemon to a pitcher and allowing it to infuse for a few hours or overnight in the refrigerator. You can also incorporate additional detoxifying ingredients like cucumber, mint, or ginger to enhance the taste and reap extra advantages.
- Consistent Intake: Make lemon water a part of your everyday regimen by sipping on it throughout the day. It can provide a refreshing and healthy option compared to sugary beverages and sodas.

Staying properly hydrated and ensuring your body is free from toxins are essential aspects of maintaining a healthy lifestyle and play a crucial role in preventing and managing infections caused by parasites. Water is crucial for cellular function, waste removal, digestive health, and immune function. Including lemon in water can boost its detoxifying properties, aid in liver function, and promote better digestion. Regularly drinking lemon water can support proper hydration and create an environment that is unfavorable for parasites.

CHAPTER 4

Herbs for Parasite Elimination

Throughout history, herbs have been utilized to address a wide range of health issues, including infections caused by parasites. They possess bioactive compounds that have the potential to hinder or eliminate parasites, enhance the immune system, and promote overall well-being. Wormwood is a highly effective herb for eliminating parasites. In this section, we will delve into the advantages, application, and techniques for preparing wormwood.

A. Wormwood

Wormwood (Artemisia absinthium) is a bitter herb known for its medicinal properties, especially in the treatment of parasitic infections. Originally found in Europe, North Africa, and Asia, this plant has now spread to various regions across the globe.

 1. Advantages and Application

- Effective Against Parasites: Wormwood possesses a variety of bioactive compounds, including sesquiterpene lactones like artemisinin, that exhibit potent antiparasitic effects. These compounds function by causing harm to the cellular membranes of the parasite, disturbing their metabolism, and preventing their reproductive capabilities.

- Boosting Immune Function: Wormwood possesses properties that can assist in regulating and fortifying the immune system, providing support for its optimal functioning. A strong immune system is essential for detecting and getting rid of unwanted organisms from the body.

- Promoting Digestive Health: The bitter compounds found in wormwood have been shown to stimulate the production of digestive juices, such as saliva, gastric acid, and bile. This supports improved digestion, nutrient absorption, and regular bowel movements, facilitating the elimination of parasites and their eggs.

- Wormwood possesses properties that can aid in reducing inflammation and oxidative stress resulting from parasitic infections, offering potential anti-inflammatory and antioxidant effects. This promotes general well-being and aids in the healing process from the harm inflicted by parasites.

- Application: Wormwood can be utilized in a variety of ways, such as in its dried herb form, as a tincture, in capsules, or brewed as a tea. It is crucial to seek the guidance of a healthcare professional when using wormwood, as this potent herb can be toxic if taken in high doses or used for an extended period of time.

 2. Methods of Preparation

- Wormwood Tea: - Ingredients: Combine 1 teaspoon of dried wormwood leaves with 1 cup of boiling water.
  - Getting Ready:
    1. Put the dried wormwood leaves in a teapot or cup.
    2. Pour hot water over the leaves.
    3. Cover and allow it to steep for 5-10 minutes.
    4. Filter the tea to separate the leaves.
    For optimal results, it is recommended to consume the tea on an empty stomach. It is recommended to consume it 1-2 times per day for a maximum duration of two weeks.
  - Note: Wormwood tea has a strong and bitter taste. If desired, a touch of honey or lemon can be added to enhance the flavor.

- Wormwood Tincture: - Ingredients: Dried leaves of the wormwood plant, 80-100 proof vodka or brandy.
  - Preparation:
    1. Fill a glass jar halfway with dried wormwood leaves.
    2. Pour the alcohol of your choice over the leaves until the jar is full.

3. Securely close the jar and place it in a cool, dark location for 4-6 weeks, giving it an occasional shake.

4. Filter the mixture using a cheesecloth or fine mesh strainer to separate the plant material.

Remember to store the tincture in a dark glass bottle.

- Dosage: Take 10-15 drops of the tincture in a small amount of water 2-3 times a day before meals. It is advisable to seek guidance from a healthcare professional regarding the correct dosage and duration.

- Wormwood Capsules: - Ingredients: Dried leaves of wormwood, capsules made of gelatin or suitable for vegetarians.

- Getting Ready:

1. Pulverize the dried wormwood leaves into a fine powder using a mortar and pestle or a coffee grinder.

2. Fill the empty capsules with the wormwood powder using a capsule-filling machine or by hand.

3. It is important to store the filled capsules in a cool, dry place.

- Administration: Usually, a recommended dosage of wormwood powder is 200-300 mg per capsule, to be taken 1-3 times daily before meals. It is important to consult with a healthcare professional to determine the appropriate dosage.

Wormwood is a potent herb known for its remarkable ability to combat parasites, making it a valuable natural solution for eradicating these unwanted organisms. It offers various advantages such as boosting the immune system, improving digestive health, and delivering anti-inflammatory and antioxidant properties. Wormwood is available in different forms, including tea, tincture, or capsules.

B. Black Walnut Hull
Black walnut hull is a potent natural remedy for parasitic infections. This ancient herbal remedy has been relied upon for generations to purify the body of unwanted organisms and harmful invaders. In this section, we will delve into the advantages and applications of black walnut hull, along with the various ways it can be prepared.

1. Advantages and Applications

- Effective against Parasites: Black walnut hull contains juglone, a powerful compound that has been found to be effective against parasites, fungi, and bacteria. Juglone has the ability to disrupt the metabolism of parasites and other pathogens, resulting in their demise and preventing their ability to reproduce.

- Abundant in Nutrients: Black walnut hull contains a variety of essential vitamins and minerals, such as vitamin C, vitamin B6, iodine, and potassium. These nutrients promote general well-being and boost the body's immune system to combat infections.

- Promoting Digestive Health: The astringent properties of black walnut hull can support the well-being of the digestive tract and aid in eliminating unwanted organisms. In addition, they enhance bile production, assisting in the process of digestion and the removal of waste.

- Boosting Immune System: The antimicrobial properties of black walnut hull aid in enhancing the efficiency of the immune system, enabling it to better detect and eliminate parasites.

- Application: Black walnut hull can be utilized in a variety of forms, such as tinctures, capsules, and powders. It is crucial to seek the guidance of a healthcare professional when using black walnut hull, particularly in higher doses or for extended periods.

 Typical Applications:
- Internal Cleansing: Black walnut hull is commonly utilized in detoxification

programs to purify the digestive tract of harmful substances and impurities.

- Topical Applications: A natural remedy that can be applied externally to address fungal infections, like athlete's foot and ringworm.

- Boosting Immunity: Consistently incorporating black walnut hull into your routine can fortify your immune system and safeguard against harmful infections.

2. Methods of Preparation

- Tincture made from the hull of the Black Walnut tree: - Components: Using fresh or dried black walnut hulls and 80-100 proof vodka or brandy.

  - Getting Ready:

    1. Put the black walnut hulls in a glass jar, filling it approximately halfway.

    2. Pour the alcohol of your choice over the hulls until the jar is full.

    3. Securely close the jar and place it in a cool, dark location for 4-6 weeks, giving it an occasional shake.

    4. Filter the mixture using a cheesecloth or fine mesh strainer to separate the plant material.

    Remember to store the tincture in a dark glass bottle.

  - Administration: Take 10-20 drops of the tincture in a small amount of water 2-3 times a day before meals. It is advisable to seek guidance from a healthcare professional regarding the correct dosage and duration.

- Black Walnut Hull Capsules: - Ingredients: Dried black walnut hulls, empty gelatin or vegetarian capsules.
  - Getting Ready:
    1. Pulverize the dried black walnut hulls into a fine powder using a mortar and pestle or a coffee grinder.
    2. Fill the empty capsules with the black walnut powder using a capsule-filling machine or by hand.
    3. It is important to store the filled capsules in a cool, dry place.
  - Administration: Usually, a recommended dosage of black walnut powder per capsule is 500-1,000 mg. It is advised to take the capsules 1-3 times a day before meals. It is important to consult with a healthcare professional to determine the appropriate dosage.

- Black Walnut Hull Tea: - Ingredients: Combine 1 teaspoon of dried black walnut hull powder with 1 cup of boiling water.
  - Getting Ready:
    1. Put the black walnut hull powder in a teapot or cup.
    2. Pour hot water over the powder.
    3. Cover and allow it to steep for 10-15 minutes.

4. Filter the tea to separate the powder.

For optimal results, it is recommended to consume the tea on an empty stomach. It is recommended to take it once or twice a day for a maximum of two weeks.
- Note: The taste of black walnut tea can be quite bitter. If desired, a touch of honey or lemon can be added to enhance the flavor.

Black walnut hull is a potent herb known for its impressive ability to combat parasites, making it a valuable natural solution for eradicating these unwanted organisms. It offers various advantages such as boosting the immune system, improving digestive health, and exerting antimicrobial properties. Black walnut hull is available in different forms, including tinctures, capsules, or tea.

C. Cloves
Cloves, known for their aromatic properties, are widely used as a spice in different culinary traditions across the globe. In addition to their culinary applications, cloves have long been valued for their healing properties, especially in addressing digestive problems and combating parasitic infections. This section delves into the advantages, application, and techniques

for preparing cloves to eliminate parasites.

1. Advantages and Application

- Powerful Properties: Cloves contain eugenol, a compound known for its strong antiparasitic, antimicrobial, and antioxidant effects. Research has demonstrated that eugenol is highly effective in preventing the growth and reproduction of various parasites, such as intestinal worms and protozoa.
- Promoting Digestive Health: Cloves have been found to stimulate digestive enzymes and support the production of gastric acids, which can help improve digestion and enhance nutrient absorption. Additionally, they possess carminative properties that aid in alleviating discomfort caused by gas, bloating, and indigestion.
- Boosting Immune Function: The powerful antioxidant properties of cloves can enhance the immune system's strength by counteracting harmful free radicals and minimizing oxidative stress. An effective immune system is crucial in defending against parasitic infections.
- Soothing Inflammation: Cloves have properties that can help soothe inflammation in the gastrointestinal tract, which can be caused by certain infections.

This can help relieve discomfort and support the healing process.
- Oral Health: Cloves are frequently utilized in dental care products because of their antibacterial properties. Using cloves or clove oil can provide relief for toothaches and gum infections caused by bacteria and parasites.
- Usage: Cloves can be utilized in different forms, such as whole cloves, ground cloves, clove oil, or capsules. Adding cloves to your diet or using them as a supplement can help promote the elimination of parasites and improve your overall well-being.

Common Uses: - Whole Cloves: Incorporate whole cloves into your cooking, particularly in savory dishes like stews, soups, and rice dishes, to enhance the flavor and enjoy their potential health benefits.
- Ground Cloves: Ground cloves are a versatile ingredient that adds a delightful aroma and numerous health benefits to your baking, spice blends, and teas.
- Clove Oil: It is important to dilute clove essential oil before using it, as it is highly concentrated. It can be used on the skin or gums, or in aromatherapy diffusers.
- Clove Capsules: Capsules containing clove supplements are readily available, with a standardized eugenol content. They offer a convenient method to

access the therapeutic advantages of cloves.

2. Methods of Preparation

- Clove Tea: - Ingredients: Combine one teaspoon of whole cloves or ground cloves with one cup of boiling water.
  - Getting Ready:
    1. Put the cloves in a teapot or cup.
    2. Pour hot water over the cloves.
    3. Cover and allow it to steep for 10-15 minutes.
    4. Filter the tea to separate the cloves.
    Enjoy the tea while it's still warm. It is recommended to consume it 1-2 times a day for a maximum of two weeks.
  - Note: The taste of clove tea is robust and full of spice. If desired, a touch of honey or lemon can be added to enhance the flavor.

- Clove Oil Infusion: - Ingredients: Whole cloves or ground cloves, carrier oil (such as olive oil or coconut oil).
  - Getting Ready:
    1. Fill a glass jar halfway with cloves, whether whole or ground.
    Step 2: Make sure the cloves are fully covered by the carrier oil.
    3. Securely close the jar and position it in a warm, sunlit area for 2-4 weeks, giving it an occasional shake.

4. Filter the oil using a cheesecloth or fine mesh strainer to separate the cloves.

5. Keep the infused oil in a dark glass bottle in a cool, dark place.

- Application: Apply the clove-infused oil directly to the abdomen or affected areas and gently massage. Additionally, it has potential applications as a mouthwash or gargle to promote oral health.

- Clove Capsules: - Ingredients: Finely ground cloves and empty gelatin or vegetarian capsules.

 - Getting Ready:

1. Fill the empty capsules with ground cloves using a capsule-filling machine or by hand.

2. It is important to store the filled capsules in a cool, dry place.

- Recommended amount: Usually, a dosage of 500-1,000 mg of ground cloves per capsule is recommended, to be taken 1-3 times a day before meals. It is important to consult with a healthcare professional to determine the appropriate dosage.

Cloves are not just a delicious spice, but also a powerful herbal remedy that offers a wide range of health benefits, including its ability to combat parasites. They have the potential to improve digestive health, strengthen the immune system, decrease inflammation, and enhance oral health. Cloves can be utilized in different ways, including tea, oil infusions, or capsules, to support the removal of parasites and promote overall health.

CHAPTER 5

Diet and Lifestyle Modifications

A. Anti-inflammatory Diet

Following a diet that helps reduce inflammation is essential for bolstering the body's innate ability to combat parasitic infections. Through the reduction of inflammation and the promotion of immune function, this dietary approach can effectively support herbal treatments and aid in the eradication of unwanted organisms. Important elements of a diet that helps reduce inflammation involve minimizing the consumption of sugar and processed foods, and instead focusing on increasing fiber intake.

1. Limiting the consumption of sugary and processed foods

Reducing the intake of sugar and processed foods is a key aspect of an anti-inflammatory diet. These foods can worsen inflammation, compromise the immune system, and create a favorable environment in the body for parasites to thrive and multiply.

- Sugar: Consuming too much refined sugars and high-fructose corn syrup can have negative effects on the immune system and contribute to inflammation. Reducing sugar intake can effectively hinder the reproduction and survival of parasites.
- Processed Foods: Consuming processed foods can lead to the intake of unhealthy fats, preservatives, artificial additives, and refined carbohydrates, which may have negative effects on our health. These ingredients have the potential to disturb the delicate balance of gut flora and increase inflammation, which can make the body more vulnerable to infections caused by parasites.

 Ways to Decrease Consumption of Sugar and Processed Foods:

- Be Mindful of Labels: Steer clear of foods containing added sugars, artificial sweeteners, and ingredients that may be a mouthful to pronounce.
- Embrace Nutritious Choices: Emphasize the inclusion of fresh fruits, vegetables, whole grains, lean proteins, and healthy fats in your diet, while minimizing the consumption of packaged and processed foods.
- Reduce Consumption of Sugary Drinks: Opt for healthier alternatives such as water, herbal teas, or infused water with

lemon or cucumber instead of sugary sodas and juices.

2. Boosting Fiber Consumption

Having a sufficient amount of dietary fiber is important for maintaining a healthy digestive system and ensuring regular bowel movements. This helps in getting rid of unwanted organisms and their waste products from the body. Fiber is essential for supporting a balanced gut microbiome, which plays a vital role in boosting immune function and promoting overall wellness.

- Soluble Fiber: Can be found in a variety of foods including oats, barley, nuts, seeds, beans, and lentils. Consuming soluble fiber can have a positive impact on digestion and nutrient absorption by creating a gel-like substance in the digestive tract when it interacts with water.
- Insoluble Fiber: Can be found in a variety of foods, including whole grains, vegetables, and fruits that have skins or seeds. Adding insoluble fiber to your diet can help increase the bulk of your stool, encourage regular bowel movements, and aid in the efficient elimination of waste from your body.

Advantages of Boosting Fiber Consumption:

- Enhanced Digestive Well-being: Fiber plays a crucial role in maintaining a healthy digestive system, aiding in the prevention of constipation and supporting regularity. This can help reduce the risk of infections caused by parasites by effectively eliminating waste and toxins from the body.
- Promotes Gut Microbiome Health: Fiber serves as a source of nourishment for beneficial gut bacteria, which are essential for maintaining a strong immune system and overall well-being.
- Feeling Satisfied and Managing Weight: Incorporating high-fiber foods into your diet can help you feel more satisfied and reduce cravings for unhealthy snacks and sweets.

Tips for Boosting Your Fiber Intake:

- Emphasize Whole Grains: Opt for whole grains like brown rice, quinoa, whole wheat, and oats over refined grains.
- Nourish Your Body with Nutrient-Rich Foods: Enhance your meals by including a diverse range of vibrant vegetables, such as leafy greens, cruciferous veggies like broccoli and cauliflower, and root vegetables like carrots and sweet potatoes.
- Incorporate Legumes and Beans: Incorporate beans, lentils, chickpeas, and peas into your soups, salads, and

stews to enjoy a nutritious boost of fiber and plant-based protein.
- Healthy Snacking: Indulge in the goodness of fresh fruits, complete with their natural skins, and savor the crunch of nutrient-packed nuts and seeds for a wholesome and fiber-rich snack.

 Practical Tips for Incorporating Dietary Changes:

- Gradual Transition: Begin by incorporating small adjustments into your diet, gradually increasing the intake of fiber-rich foods while simultaneously reducing the consumption of sugar and processed foods.
- Meal Planning: Plan nutritious meals that incorporate a range of fiber sources to help you meet your daily fiber requirements.
- Hydration: It is important to stay well-hydrated by drinking plenty of water throughout the day. This helps to support healthy digestion and ensures that fiber functions properly.

A diet that prioritizes reducing sugar and processed foods while increasing fiber intake is crucial for bolstering the body's innate defenses against parasitic infections. Through reducing inflammation, enhancing digestive health, and boosting the immune system, this dietary method can work alongside herbal remedies to aid in the successful eradication of parasites.

Fasting and Detox Programs
Engaging in fasting and detox programs can provide valuable support for the body's innate detoxification mechanisms and boost the efficacy of treatments for parasitic infections. This section delves into the concepts of intermittent fasting, juice fasting, and herbal detox teas, emphasizing their potential benefits in eliminating parasites.

1. Intermittent Fasting

Intermittent fasting (IF) is a dietary approach that involves alternating between periods of eating and fasting. There are different patterns of IF, such as the 16/8 method (fasting for 16 hours and having an 8-hour eating window) or the 5:2 method (eating normally for five days and significantly reducing calorie intake for two non-consecutive days). Intermittent fasting has become increasingly popular due to its potential health benefits that extend beyond weight loss. It has been associated with improvements in metabolic health, a reduction in inflammation, and support for cellular repair processes.

Advantages of Intermittent Fasting for Eliminating Parasites:

- Cellular Autophagy: Fasting stimulates cellular autophagy, a natural process in which cells eliminate damaged components, including harmful organisms and infected cells.
- Regulation of Gut Microbiota: Intermittent fasting can support a well-balanced gut bacteria, which plays a vital role in immune function and protection against harmful organisms.
- Improved Immune Response: Fasting has been found to enhance immune function by reducing inflammation and oxidative stress, which can aid the body in fighting off parasitic infections more effectively.

Helpful Suggestions for Intermittent Fasting:

- Take it Easy: Start off with shorter fasting periods and gradually increase the duration as your body gets used to it.
- Remember to keep yourself properly hydrated: Make sure to stay well-hydrated by drinking plenty of water throughout your fasting periods. This will help support your body's detoxification process and keep you properly hydrated.
- Optimal Nutrition: Prioritize consuming foods that are rich in nutrients during

your designated eating periods to enhance your overall well-being and boost your immune system.

2. Juice Fasting

During a juice fast, individuals consume only fresh fruit and vegetable juices for a specific duration, which can vary from a few days to several weeks. Drinks are packed with vitamins, minerals, antioxidants, and enzymes, which can aid in detoxification and provide vital nutrients while allowing the digestive system to rest from solid foods.

Benefits of Juice Fasting for Eliminating Parasites:

- Enhanced Nutritional Value: Fresh juices offer a rich source of vitamins, minerals, and antioxidants that bolster immune function and facilitate detoxification.
- Staying Hydrated: Drinking juices can help keep your body hydrated, which is important for eliminating toxins and waste products, including harmful organisms.
- Creating an Unfavorable Environment: Numerous fruits and vegetables possess properties that create an environment less conducive for parasites to thrive.

Practical Tips for a Juice Cleanse:

- Opt for organic produce: Select fruits and vegetables that are grown organically to reduce pesticide exposure and increase nutrient content.
- Diverse Selection of Juices: Incorporate a wide range of fruits and vegetables into your juices to guarantee a rich array of nutrients.
- Stay Mindful of Energy Levels: Pay attention to your body's signals and take breaks when necessary while juice fasting to promote a sense of vitality and overall health.

3. Herbal Cleanse Teas

Herbal detox teas are a combination of medicinal herbs that are renowned for their ability to cleanse and purify the body. These teas commonly contain herbs like dandelion root, burdock root, milk thistle, and ginger. These herbs are known to promote liver health, aid digestion, and assist in the removal of toxins from the body.

Benefits of Herbal Detox Teas for Eliminating Parasites:

- Supporting Liver Health: Herbs such as dandelion root and milk thistle can aid in the detoxification process of the liver,

assisting in the removal of toxins and waste products from the body.
- Digestive Aid: Ginger and other digestive herbs can enhance digestion, alleviate bloating, and assist in eliminating unwanted organisms and their byproducts.
- Beneficial Effects Against Parasites: Certain herbs found in detox teas, like wormwood and black walnut hull, possess properties that can help combat parasites, making them a valuable addition to parasite elimination protocols.

Practical Tips for Herbal Detox Teas:

- Premium Ingredients: Opt for top-notch, organic herbal teas to guarantee purity and maximize effectiveness.
- Brewing Time: Adhere to the suggested brewing durations to fully extract the potential benefits of the herbs.
- Important Note: It is advisable to seek guidance from a healthcare professional prior to consuming herbal detox teas, particularly if you have any pre-existing health conditions or are currently on medication.

Exploring various fasting and detox programs, such as intermittent fasting, juice fasting, and herbal detox teas, can provide valuable support for the body's detoxification processes and help eliminate parasites. These strategies can assist in minimizing inflammation, bolstering immune function, and enhancing overall health and well-being.

D. Maintaining a Balanced pH

In order to maintain a well-balanced pH and enhance the body's innate ability to combat parasitic infections, it is essential to prioritize alkaline foods and limit the consumption of acidic foods. This section delves into the importance of maintaining a proper pH balance through dietary choices and how it can affect one's overall well-being.

C. Maintaining a Proper pH Balance

Ensuring a well-regulated pH level in the body is crucial for maintaining overall well-being and a strong immune system. The pH scale is used to determine the acidity or alkalinity of a substance. It ranges from 0, which indicates high acidity, to 14, which indicates high alkalinity. A pH of 7 is considered neutral. The pH level of the human body is carefully maintained within a narrow range of 7.35 to 7.45, creating a slightly alkaline environment.

1. Foods with an Alkaline pH

Alkaline foods are known for their ability to have a pH above 7, which is thought to be beneficial in maintaining or restoring the body's optimal pH balance. These foods are usually packed with essential minerals like potassium, calcium, magnesium, and phosphorus. Here are some examples:

- Leafy Greens: Spinach, kale, Swiss chard, and other leafy greens provide a wide range of alkalizing minerals and phytonutrients that can be beneficial for your health.
- Vegetables: Broccoli, cabbage, cucumber, celery, and bell peppers are rich in alkaline-forming nutrients and fiber.
- Fruits: Citrus fruits (lemons, limes), watermelon, bananas, and berries are packed with vitamins and antioxidants, making them a healthy choice.
- Root Vegetables: Sweet potatoes, carrots, beets, and radishes are packed with nutrients and help maintain a balanced pH level in the body.
- Nuts and Seeds: Almonds, flaxseeds, and pumpkin seeds are nutritious options that contribute to a balanced diet. They are rich in healthy fats, protein, and fiber, which are beneficial for overall health.

 Advantages of Consuming Alkaline Foods:

- Promotes Detoxification: Alkaline foods play a crucial role in supporting the proper functioning of the liver and kidneys, which are vital for eliminating toxins and waste products from the body.
- Reduces Inflammation: Numerous alkaline foods possess properties that can combat inflammation, providing relief from the inflammation commonly linked to parasitic infections.
- Supports Bone Health: Alkaline foods are known for their calcium and magnesium content, which play a vital role in promoting bone health and keeping your skeletal system strong.

 Practical Tips for Incorporating Alkaline Foods:

- Maintain a Well-Balanced Diet: Strive to incorporate a generous portion of alkaline-forming vegetables and fruits on your plate during every meal.
- Healthy Smoothies: Add leafy greens and alkaline fruits to your smoothies for a nutritious and alkalizing boost.
- Enjoy Nuts and Seeds as a Snack: Opt for almonds, pumpkin seeds, or sunflower seeds as a delicious and nourishing snack choice.

 2. Steer Clear of Acidic Foods

Foods with a pH below 7, known as acidic foods, can potentially lead to increased acidity in the body if consumed excessively. These types of foods usually consist of:

- Processed Foods: Fast foods, packaged snacks, and sugary treats frequently include artificial additives and preservatives that may contribute to acidity levels.
- Consuming large quantities of red meat, poultry, and dairy products can lead to increased acidity levels.
- Processed Carbohydrates and Sweeteners: Consuming white bread, pasta, pastries, and sugary beverages can cause fluctuations in blood sugar levels and contribute to an acidic environment.
- Caffeine and Alcohol: Consuming excessive amounts of coffee, tea, energy drinks, and alcoholic beverages can disrupt the pH balance due to their acidic nature.

Impact of Acidic Foods:

- Inflammation: Consuming acidic foods can potentially worsen symptoms of infections caused by parasites and weaken the immune system.
- Digestive Discomfort: Consuming acidic foods may lead to various digestive

problems, including acid reflux, bloating, and indigestion.
- Mineral Depletion: Certain types of food with acidic properties have the potential to extract important minerals such as calcium, magnesium, and potassium from the body, which can have an impact on one's overall health.

 Helpful Suggestions for Decreasing Acidic Foods:

- Balance: It's important to find a balance when consuming acidic foods, ensuring that you also incorporate alkaline foods into your diet.
- Organic Market: Opt for whole grains, lean proteins, and plant-based sources of protein to reduce acidity levels.
- Proper hydration: It is important to ensure that you drink an adequate amount of water to support the elimination of acidic byproducts and to keep your body properly hydrated.

Ensuring a well-balanced pH level by consuming a diet that includes plenty of alkaline foods and limiting acidic foods can help bolster the body's innate ability to fend off parasitic infections. Foods with an alkaline nature offer vital nutrients, aid in detoxification, and contribute to reducing inflammation, thereby creating an environment that is less favorable for the growth of parasites. By incorporating a greater variety of alkaline-forming foods into your daily diet and reducing the consumption of acidic foods, you can improve the balance of pH in your body, support your overall well-being, and boost your body's natural ability to eliminate parasites effectively.

CHAPTER 6

Methods and Protocols

A. Cleansing Protocols

Detoxification protocols are structured methods created to aid the body's natural cleansing processes and improve the efficacy of treatments against parasitic infections. This section delves into detailed protocols for parasite cleansing and colon cleansing, providing an overview of their methods and potential advantages.

1. Protocol for Cleansing Parasites

A protocol for eliminating parasites from the body includes incorporating different herbs, making dietary adjustments, and utilizing supportive therapies. This protocol is frequently incorporated into a comprehensive approach to health and well-being, with the goal of enhancing digestion, strengthening the immune system, and alleviating symptoms commonly associated with infections caused by parasites.

Elements of a Protocol for Cleansing Parasites:

- Natural Remedies: Certain herbs like wormwood, black walnut hull, cloves, and garlic are often sought after for their ability to combat parasites. These herbs are commonly used in specific formulations or combinations to address various types of parasites.
- Dietary Modifications: Adopting a diet that focuses on fresh fruits, vegetables, lean proteins, and whole grains, while steering clear of sugar, processed foods, and allergens, can help create an environment that is less favorable for parasites.
- Hydration: Staying well-hydrated by drinking ample water and herbal teas can aid in eliminating harmful substances and promoting the body's natural detoxification processes.
- Supportive Therapies: Practices like intermittent fasting, sauna therapy, and exercise can help improve detoxification and promote overall health while undergoing a cleanse.
- Duration: Parasite cleanse protocols usually range from a few weeks to a couple of months, depending on the seriousness of the infection and how individuals respond to treatment.

 Advantages of a Protocol for Cleansing Parasites:

- Relieving Symptoms: Decreasing the presence of parasites can help alleviate common symptoms like bloating, gas, diarrhea, and fatigue that are often associated with parasitic infections.
- Enhanced Digestive Health: Boosting digestive function and maintaining a healthy balance of gut flora can improve nutrient absorption and promote overall digestive well-being.
- Improved Immune Function: By eliminating parasites, the immune system can better allocate its resources to defending against other pathogens and maintaining overall health, resulting in enhanced immune function.

 Practical Tips for an Effective Cleanse Protocol:

- Consultation: Seek guidance from a healthcare professional or naturopathic doctor who specializes in dealing with parasitic infections. They will be able to create a personalized cleanse protocol that suits your individual requirements.
- Please adhere to the instructions provided: Adhere to the prescribed dosage instructions for herbal supplements and protocols to guarantee both safety and efficacy.
- Keep an eye on any changes in your symptoms: Be mindful of any shifts in symptoms and your overall state of

health while undergoing the cleanse, and make any necessary adjustments to the protocol.

2. Cleansing the Colon

Colon cleansing, also referred to as colonic irrigation or colonic hydrotherapy, is a therapeutic procedure that focuses on purifying the colon by removing accumulated waste, toxins, and potentially harmful substances. While a subject of debate among medical professionals, supporters argue that colon cleansing may have potential benefits for digestive health, alleviating constipation, and aiding in detoxification.

Different Approaches to Colon Cleansing:

- Colon Hydrotherapy: Involves the gentle cleansing of the colon using water, which helps eliminate waste and toxins from the body. This procedure is typically carried out by skilled experts in a medical environment.
- Enemas: A procedure that individuals can perform on themselves by infusing water or a solution into the rectum. This helps stimulate bowel movements and cleanse the colon.
- Detoxification Methods: Some dietary plans or fasting routines may incorporate elements that encourage bowel

movements and the removal of toxins from the colon.

 Advantages of Colon Cleansing:

- Enhanced Digestive Function: Colon cleansing can help alleviate symptoms such as constipation, bloating, and gas by effectively eliminating impacted fecal matter and toxins from the colon.
- Support for Detoxification: By helping to eliminate waste and toxins, colon cleansing can assist in supporting the body's overall detoxification processes.
- Possible Health Advantages: Some supporters claim that colon cleansing may enhance overall health and boost immune function by reducing the presence of toxins in the body.

B. Supportive Therapies
To enhance parasite cleansing protocols and encourage overall detoxification, a range of supportive therapies can be incorporated into a comprehensive health regimen.

Supportive therapies are additional treatments that can boost the effectiveness of parasite cleansing protocols. They work by aiding in detoxification, enhancing circulation, and promoting relaxation.

1. Rectal Irrigation

Enemas are a method used to cleanse and remove waste material from the colon by introducing liquid through the rectum. This therapy is effective in relieving constipation, eliminating impacted fecal matter, and promoting detoxification processes.

Different Types of Enemas:

- Water Enemas: A widely used method that entails the introduction of purified water into the colon to promote bowel movements and purify the lower digestive tract.
- Coffee Enemas: Coffee enemas are thought to promote bile flow and improve liver detoxification processes. They are commonly utilized in detoxification protocols to promote comprehensive cleansing.
- Herbal Enemas: Utilize herbs with distinct properties (such as anti-inflammatory or antimicrobial) to promote digestive health and detoxification.

Advantages of Enemas for Cleansing Parasites:

- Colon Cleansing: Enemas can assist in eliminating accumulated waste, toxins,

and other substances from the colon, promoting a healthier environment that is less favorable for certain organisms.
- Support for Natural Detoxification: Enemas can help stimulate bowel movements and promote waste elimination, which can support the body's natural detoxification processes.
- Relief from Symptoms: Enemas can help alleviate discomfort in the abdomen, bloating, and gas that are commonly experienced with certain infections.

2. Utilizing Castor Oil Packs

Castor oil packs involve applying a cloth soaked in castor oil to the skin, usually over the abdomen. This therapy is thought to aid in detoxification, decrease inflammation, and facilitate healing.

Advantages of Castor Oil Packs:

- Supporting Liver Function: Castor oil packs are believed to enhance liver detoxification pathways, aiding in the removal of toxins and metabolic waste products, including those associated with certain organisms.
- Soothing Effects: The use of castor oil packs can provide relief from inflammation in the abdomen and promote a sense of comfort in digestion.

- Promoting Relaxation and Stress Reduction: The comforting and calming effects of castor oil packs can contribute to a sense of relaxation, which can be advantageous for enhancing overall well-being and managing stress.

3. Infrared Sauna Therapy

Using infrared light, infrared sauna therapy can effectively heat the body and stimulate sweating, which aids in detoxification. This therapy is distinct from traditional saunas as it utilizes infrared wavelengths to deeply penetrate tissues, promoting cellular detoxification.
Advantages of Infrared Sauna Therapy:

- Detoxification: Sweating induced by infrared sauna therapy aids in the elimination of toxins, heavy metals, and metabolic waste products through the skin, promoting overall detoxification.
- Enhanced Circulation: Infrared heat facilitates vasodilation and boosts blood flow, which improves the supply of oxygen and nutrients to tissues while assisting in the elimination of toxins.
- Promoting Relaxation and Reducing Stress: The soothing warmth and calming effects of infrared sauna therapy can help alleviate stress, foster relaxation, and contribute to a sense of overall mental and physical well-being.

Enemas, castor oil packs, and infrared sauna therapy can be beneficial complementary therapies that may improve the efficacy of parasite cleansing protocols and promote overall detoxification. These therapies support the body's natural processes of cleansing and detoxification, which can have a positive impact on digestive health and overall well-being.

THE END